TALK TO SOMEONE:

A Talk With Someone Eases You from Depression and Anxiety

By

Dr Sharon Black

Table of Content

- **Inquire whether they want to speak with you**
- **Remind them that they are Important**
- **Tell them you are Aware of their Situation (If You Really Do)**
- **Remind Them It's OK to Feel The Way They Feel**
- **Educate Them It's Alright to Feel That Way**
- **Assure them that they are not Defective or Weak**
- **Insist on the Fact that there is Hope**

CHAPTER FOUR

Know the Suicide Warning Signs

CONCLUSION

INTRODUCTION

Because major depression is one of the most common mental health conditions in the world, someone you know or love is likely to be affected. Knowing how to talk to someone who is depressed can be a really helpful method to help them.

While reaching out to someone who is depressed will not heal them, it will remind them that they are not alone. When you're depressed, this can be difficult to believe, but it can be really beneficial in a crisis.

I'll assist you in gaining a better knowledge of sadness and anxiety, as well as common and often unnoticed symptoms. We'll look at some more negative effects of depression before moving on to some tactics you can employ to help someone who is depressed or anxious. It's critical to have a basic understanding of depression and anxiety in order to successfully support someone who suffers from it.

Both depression and anxiety have physical components and involve neurotransmitter and hormone abnormalities, therefore it's a physiological imbalance. Now, our ideas, feelings, and surroundings can all contribute to that physiological imbalance, but it's vital to remember that there's also a physical component. So, just as you wouldn't advise someone to get over the virus, you won't be able to tell them to get over their depression since it's not that simple. Anxiety and depression are caused by a variety of factors, and many people feel both at the same time. They may be depressed and anxious about whether their depression will worsen, whether people will reject them, and so on. They may be nervous and feel helpless and hopeless in dealing with the issues that are causing them anxiety, leading to exhaustion and depression. As a result, we frequently see these two phenomena occur together. Let's start with a definition of depression.

CHAPTER ONE
SYMPTOMS

For at least two weeks, people with depression have either a low or sad mood, a loss of pleasure, or a lack of colour or sensation in their day. However, there is a condition known as persistent depressive disorder, which can linger for two years or longer. It's critical to determine if someone is depressed or simply has the feeling that they don't feel much of anything, that they are numb all of the time, or that life is devoid of colour. That does not have to be the case, therefore that is one symptom.

Another indication of depression is Sleep disturbances. Many people who are depressed are exhausted, so they want to sleep a lot. However, they don't get good sleep, and they may fall asleep at the wrong time and wake up in the middle of the night, or they may go to bed at a reasonable time but still wake up in the middle of the night and can't fall back asleep. Because sleep disruptions are so widespread, it's crucial to understand that serotonin is one possible neurochemical linked in depression. Others, such as norepinephrine and dopamine, might induce depressed symptoms, but serotonin is broken down to make melatonin, which helps us go asleep. People who are depressed, especially if their depression is caused by a serotonin imbalance, often have trouble getting quality restful sleep, and it's not necessarily because of anything they're doing; it could be because of that imbalance, because those sleep changes cause changes in their circadian rhythms, and their body may start losing its normal internal clock and not knowing when it's sleepy, when it's awake. As a result, oestrogen, testosterone, and progesterone may no longer be needed.

Depression affects people's eating habits. Many people with depression prefer high-fat, high-sugar foods because they induce serotonin and dopamine to be released. However, other people who are depressed have no appetite at all; in either case, the body is likely not obtaining all of the other essential nutrients. So, while dietary changes might be a symptom of depression, they can also cause depression.

Another symptom of depression is a lack of energy. People's energy levels are affected when they don't get enough sleep, when they don't eat enough, and when their serotonin, dopamine, and norepinephrine are depleted, hence many people have low energy. But there can be a variety of reasons for that, psychomotor retardation is a clinical word for slowing it feels like everything they're doing is in a wind tunnel and it's simply tougher and takes more energy and effort for them to do things, and it's not just them who notice it.

Another common symptom is Irritability. When people are gloomy, hopeless, powerless, or fatigued, there's a small voice in the back of their primordial brain telling them they don't have a lot of energy and are vulnerable right now. And when people feel vulnerable, they are more likely to fight or flee, which is why irritability is common among depressed people. It's their body's way of telling them they don't have the energy to fight right now, or to deal with anything else.

Guilt is common in people with depression because they don't want to be depressed or exhausted all of the time. They feel guilty for not being able to do the things they think they should, which adds to their sense of hopelessness and helplessness when they tell themselves they should, but can't.

Another common symptom of depression is difficulty concentrating, which is one of the clinical symptoms you may be familiar with. When people don't get enough sleep, adenosine, a consequence of brain activity, builds up in the brain, contributing to daytime exhaustion and making it difficult to concentrate. Dopamine and norepinephrine are two of our attention hormones, and as I previously stated, in people who are depressed, all three of these chemicals, serotonin, dopamine, and norepinephrine, are frequently out of action. Because when one loses their balance, it brings their friends with them, people may find it difficult to concentrate. Concentration requires energy, and if you don't have any, it'll be more difficult to concentrate, even if you've been sleeping well. These are the clinical criteria for depression, and they're found in the DSM. However, we also encounter persons with depression who have more pain and stiffness. So, if you're sleeping a lot and don't have the energy to walk around, you'll start to feel stiffer. You're going to have to start having more aches and pains since you're probably not using correct ergonomics whether you're sitting in front of the TV or resting in bed, which causes stiffness. Furthermore, serotonin is one of our neurochemicals involved in pain perception, and when serotonin levels are low, pain perception increases, and we begin to feel more pain that is genuine, not imagined.

CHAPTER TWO
DEPRESSION AND ANXIETY

Remember how I said they frequently co-occur? Anxiety is one of them. Anxiety is defined as a feeling of being tense or on edge the majority of the time. We call generalised anxiety worrying about a range of topics most of the time. It's not something they choose to do; they're not saying, "Hey, I want to worry about this or that!" There's something in our brain called the default mode network; it's sort of our autopilot, and people with generalised anxiety often have their default mode network take on a life of its own, constantly telling them about things that could go wrong. In persons with generalised anxiety and chronic post-traumatic or complicated post-traumatic stress disorder, the amygdala (our brain's fear centre) is larger and more active. As a result, it's critical to appreciate that they are not choosing to be concerned about everything. They have what Linehan refers to as a monkey mind every time they sit down, and those thoughts just start popping up and it feels like they're continuously inundated by them. When you're worried, it's difficult to concentrate because your brain is secreting cortisol, glutamate, and norepinephrine to give you the energy you need to fight or flee. This is not the time to concentrate.

They have sleep disturbances, and, like depressive individuals, they may be unable to sleep at all, have insomnia, or be unable to stay asleep, and they may be exhausted and tired all of the time because, guess what, they are always revving their engine. Because of their anxiousness, they are continually expending energy and being pumped up or revved up, which is draining.

They may experience increased pain, just like persons who are depressed. They've discovered that when people have anxiety, their serotonin levels are often too high. Increased glutamate or norepinephrine levels, among other factors, can produce anxiety.
However, people with anxiety typically experience heightened discomfort, which can be due to a neurochemical imbalance or because they're tense all of the time, just like when you work out and your muscles get sore. Muscle pain occurs when you are always tight. People with anxiety are more likely to have tmj, which

causes them to grind their teeth at night, causing them to wake up with pain in their teeth, jaw, and ears, which can lead to increased irritability, problems sleeping, and even worry about what's causing it. Anxious people frequently feel stomach ache and, in some cases, diarrhoea.

Other negative effects of sadness and anxiety
When people are in a state of fight or flight, the brain says, "Hey!" and reduces libido. It's not the right moment to start a family, thus the sex hormones react differently. When people are depressed, they just do not have the energy to do anything. When cortisol, our stress hormone, is high, our immunity suffers, and we notice that people's immunity is compromised in both depression and anxiety. We also know that persons with depression frequently experience systemic inflammation, causing their immune systems to become overactive.
Inflammation is aided by cortisol. Cortisol is generally an anti-inflammatory hormone, but it loses its ability to control inflammation when exposed to it on a long-term basis. As a result, inflammation goes wild, and when inflammation goes awry, we observe greater

disease and despair. More pain, as well as autoimmune flare-ups, are possible outcomes.

As well as wrath, guilt, despair, anxiety, grief, and, as previously said, poor memory. Well, I guess I didn't particularly specify weak recall when I mentioned concentration. We can't remember stuff when we can't concentrate. If you're not concentrating on something, such as reading a book or watching a movie, you won't recall what's said, and people with weak memory have trouble concentrating. They frequently forget things and make mistakes, which can make them feel guilty, awful, and lead other people to become upset with them. For instance, if you're in a relationship with someone who suffers from melancholy or anxiety and is prone to forgetfulness, Is this something they're deliberately doing? Is it possible that they are being rude, or is it more probable that they simply don't remember? They are attempting to concentrate but are unable to do so, and what can you do if they are unable to concentrate? Hint: write it down, send them push alerts, or put it wherever they can see it so they don't have to store it in their heads.

Anaemia, which is caused by an iron shortage, can create symptoms that are comparable to both despair and anxiety. Malnutrition can result in more than just an iron shortage. But deficiency in a variety of other vitamins and minerals can keep the body from being able to break down the food that you eat.

Low vitamin D has long been associated with low energy and depressive symptoms and even seasonal affective disorder hypo, which means not enough or hyper too much thyroid can mimic depression or anxiety and hypo or hypo hyper thyroid can happen at any point in life it can happen to children as well as in old people who have never had a problem with it in their life, and then all of a sudden at 65 they're diagnosed with hypothyroid and need to take a supplement but all of these are pretty easily addressed if they're diagnosed.

Circadian Rhythm Disorders can also cause anxiety or sadness because when your circadian rhythms are disrupted, everything else is disrupted as well. Circadian rhythms control your immune system, neurotransmitter production, sleep, appetite, libido, and so on. If someone's sleep becomes disrupted for whatever reason, it's crucial to determine whether this is the cause or a source of their symptoms, which may include obstructive sleep apnea.

Depression and anxiety can be brought on by sleep apnea. When people stop breathing repeatedly during the night, it deprives their brain of oxygen and wakes them up several times throughout the night, often hundreds of times. This means they aren't getting enough sleep, which might lead to sadness. Although it can cause stress and worry in some people, obstructive sleep apnea is closely linked to depression in the general population. Obstructive sleep apnea is also considerably more common in those with a history of trauma and a diagnosis of ptsd or cptsd, so if someone has that diagnosis, it's critical to check for sleep apnea as well. If you're treating low testosterone or oestrogen, remember that if the body is stressed, if the brain believes that the body doesn't have enough energy, that the situation is helpless and dismal, or that there's too much threat, the levels of gonadal hormones will change. Now, I don't want anyone to get too worked up about this since it's one of those things that can happen but isn't usually the cause of people's symptoms.

You can make recommendations, but you can't repair them; it'll be up to them to fix themselves, and you're like, "OK, OK," but it's also crucial to remember if they're suffering from depression, anxiety, or both. Their plums are drained, and the prospect of doing anything else may be too much for them. It's critical to detect or seek for incremental changes if they've been down for a time, even a month. Depression and anxiety are frequently accompanied with a sense of hopelessness and helplessness over time.If you're in a relationship with someone who is depressed or anxious, be assertive and honest with them. Make sure you don't come across as blaming when you say it.

CHAPTER THREE

What should you say to a depressed person?

Tell them how much you care.

Avoid being deterred by concerns about speaking the "wrong" thing. Too many people suffering from clinical depression feel isolated, which exacerbates their symptoms. 1 If you're stumped for words, simply say that—and let your friend know you're there for them.

When you want to say more but are having trouble expressing yourself, there are a few things you may do. There are also certain statements that may be beneficial to someone who is depressed.

"I care" is a two-word phrase that can mean a lot to someone who feels like the world is against them. This message can be conveyed with a hug or a light touch of the hand. The most essential thing is to reach out and tell them how much they mean to you.

While you may initially feel embarrassed and unsure, remember that whatever you say does not need to be meaningful or poetic. Simply put, it should be something that originates from a place of love.

Educate Them You've Arrived to Assist Them

Depression might make you feel as if no one understands or cares enough to try to grasp what you're going through, which can be isolating and burdensome.

People who are depressed prefer to retreat, according to research, so reaching out to a buddy in need is a vital first step. If your buddy isn't ready to discuss, continue to encourage them by spending time with them and checking in on them on a frequent basis, whether in person, over the phone, or via text.

It can be incredibly soothing to tell a buddy that you would be there for them every step of the way when you reach out to them.You may not know exactly what this would entail at first, but just telling their friend that you are someone they can rely on can be really beneficial.

Inquire about how you can assist.

Depression puts a lot of strain on the person who is suffering from it, both physically and mentally, therefore there are probably a lot of things you can do to help them recover.

It's also possible that your friend's melancholy has left them so exhausted and depressed that they don't know what kind of help to seek.

Prepare a few specific suggestions, such as the following:

Are you in need of assistance with cleaning or grocery shopping?

Do you want to have some company for a while?

Do you want me to accompany you to your doctor's appointments?

It can be beneficial to be specific about both the time and the activity. "Could I come over on Saturday morning and do some yard work for you?" for example, instead of "Is there anything I can do for you?"

Also keep in mind that the assistance you believe a buddy requires may not be the same as what they consider to be beneficial. Make a suggestion—and then listen.

Depression can make it difficult to do everyday duties and fulfil other obligations. Giving someone who is depressed actual, practical support might be a terrific approach to help them.

Encourage them to seek medical advice.

Treatments for depression are a vital element of recovering from depression, yet many people are ashamed of their disease or sceptical that treatment will help.

If your friend hasn't seen a doctor yet, urge them to do so and tell them that asking for help is perfectly OK. If your friend is already visiting a doctor, volunteer to assist with medicine pick-up and keeping appointments on time.

Inquire whether they want to speak with you.

The most crucial thing you can do for a sad buddy is to simply listen sympathetically while they talk about what's hurting them, allowing them to release pent-up emotions.

Make an effort to pay attention without interrupting. We all want to help individuals we care about, and we frequently provide fast fixes to alleviate our own emotions of powerlessness.People who are depressed often just need to chat without having their conversation hijacked by well-intentioned counsel.

Remind them that they are Important

If you can honestly tell your friend how much they mean to you and others, you can help them appreciate their worth and value.

When someone is suffering from depression, letting them know that they are essential in your life can go a long way.

Tell them you are aware of their situation (If You Really Do)

Before you say "I understand," double-check what you actually do. Have you ever been depressed in a clinically serious way? If you have, it may be comforting to your buddy to know that you have been through what they are going through and that things can get better. Keep in mind, however, that there are numerous varieties of depression, and even if you have had clinical depression, your experience may have been very different from what your buddy is experiencing.

If you've had a bad case of the blues, on the other hand, your friend might think you're making light of their situation by comparing it to yours. In this case, it would be best to simply admit that you don't understand exactly what they are going through, but that you care about them and want to try. Often, the best words to say are, "I don't understand, but I really want to."

Remind Them It's OK to Feel The Way They Feel

Even if your friend's problems may seem minor to you, resist the urge to judge or come up with simple solutions. The biochemical imbalances associated with depression are what is driving how bad your friend feels about certain situations—not necessarily the situations themselves.

Instead, let them know that you are sorry that they are feeling so badly and adopt an attitude of acceptance that this is how their depression is affecting them.

In this circumstance, it's better to simply confess that you don't fully understand their situation, but that you care about them and want to help. "I don't understand, but I truly want to," is often the best thing to say.

Educate Them It's Alright to Feel That Way

Resist the impulse to pass judgement or offer simplistic solutions to your friend's difficulties, even if they appear insignificant to you. It's the physiological imbalances linked with depression that are causing your friend's distress in particular situations, not the conditions themselves.

Instead, express your regret for their distress and cultivate an attitude of acceptance that this is how their melancholy manifests itself.It may take some time for your buddy to feel better if they have only recently started taking drugs or attending counselling.

Antidepressants, like antibiotics for strep throat, can take a long time to modify the chemistry in the brain (sometimes upwards of eight weeks or longer). During this time, the most important thing for your friend is to know that you will be there for them throughout their therapy, not quick fixes.

Assure them that they aren't defective or weak.

Those suffering from depression may feel helpless or as if something is wrong with them. While depression is a medical condition, persons who suffer from it may believe it is a character weakness.Reassure your friend that depression is a medical condition caused by a biochemical imbalance in the brain, not a sign of weakness. Fighting back requires a lot of strength, therefore they're probably much stronger than they think they are.

Depression is a prevalent mental health problem that can strike anyone at any time. Remind your loved one that their sentiments are not their fault and that they are capable, strong, and resilient.

Insist on the fact that there is hope.

You can reassure your buddy that they have a legitimate illness while simultaneously assuring them that there is hope, because depression, like any other medical illness, is treatable. Your acquaintance has a very good chance of feeling normal again with the help of meds and therapy.

When the Best Intentions Go Astray.

It's possible that even if you say everything "right," your friend will still be upset with you. Every person is an individual with their own thoughts and feelings, and sadness is characterised by being angry and upset.

People will sometimes lash out at others who are attempting to help them because they are in pain and don't know where to concentrate their negative emotions. Anyone in the vicinity becomes an easy target.

If this occurs, try not to take it too seriously. Maintain your composure and do everything you can to love and support your friend in any way they will allow.

CHAPTER FOUR
Know the Suicide Warning Signs

Suicide is a significant risk for persons suffering from depression. Even if you say and do everything you can to aid your friend, they may still have suicidal thoughts and feelings. Always be on the watch for suicide warning signs and know when to seek help.

Some warning indicators to look out for:

- When it comes to wanting to die, there's a lot of talk about it.
- Expressing their feelings of being a burden to others
- Extreme feelings of hopelessness and sadness
- Withdrawal from friends and family
- Mood fluctuations that occur suddenly
- Making a will or giving away possessions
- Making vague claims about whether or not they will be present in the future
- Suicide or having a suicide plot should be discussed openly.

- Suicide attempts in the past

If you notice suicidal warning signals in a loved one, chat with them and ask them to speak with a mental health professional. When there is an immediate danger, you should remove unsafe things from the house, make sure they aren't left alone, and get medical care right away.

CONCLUSION

Asking your buddy if they are depressed is often the simplest way to start a conversation. Don't make light of your friend's feelings by accusing, threatening, or blaming them. Tell them you care and that you're available to chat about it if they want.

Demonstrate your support, look for ways to assist, and remind them that there are effective treatments available. Encourage them to get help from a mental health professional and keep an eye out for indicators of suicide behavior or ideation.

www.ingramcontent.com/pod-product-compliance
Lightning Source LLC
LaVergne TN
LVHW052113160826
845678LV00015B/3532